SEIZING THE KINGDOM ON HEALING

by B. Mae Morris

I0441187

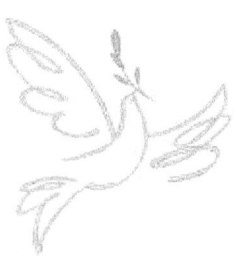

Published by: A Bridge Builder Publishing

Book Design and layout: Author

Cover by: Oxygen Ministries

First Printing, 2014

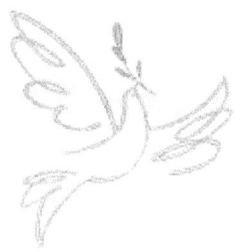

Mercy and truth meet together,
Righteousness and peace kiss each other.
Truth springs out of the earth,
Righteousness looks down from heaven.
The Lord will indeed give what is good
And our land will yield her increase.
Psalms 85: 10-12

Dedicated to the Christian believers seeking God in their sickness and have not yet received healing.
WE CARE: abridgebuilder@gmail.com

Receiving the St. Matthew award by Northwest Harvest in Seattle Washington, Bonnie has always had a heart for the needs of others. She is as passionate for the needs of your health as she has been in the teaching and evangelizing ministry.

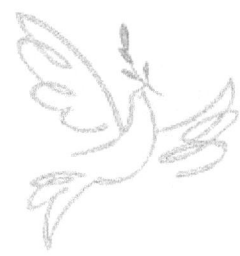

CONTENTS

INTRODUCTION

CHAPTER 1:   GOD'S MEDICINE CABINET

CHAPTER 2:   THE HELP OF SCIENCE

CHAPTER 3:   SALT 'N OIL

CHAPTER 4:   PRIESTHOOD OF THE BELIEVER

CHAPTER 5:   THE BEST OF THE BEST

SEIZING THE KINDOM ON HEALING

Introduction

Our mission is to see the body of Christ healed; to educate, and with wisdom, apply what we teach.

This book is a manual for your use to help accomplish our mission. It comes bathed in prayer to meet the needs of God's people for healing in this, and future generations. Healing for the body is a part of the wonderful grace of God!

Many people seek money, or status or material possessions, but the Bible tells us there is something more important we should seek. That something is "WISDOM".

Proverbs 4:7 *Wisdom is the principal thing; therefore get wisdom: and with all thy getting get understanding.* The source of all wisdom is God, and He will share it with us if we ask.

James 1:5 *If any of you lack wisdom, let him ask of God, that gives to all men liberally, and upbraids not; and it shall be given him.*

We like to teach about healing. Education is good and we should make use of it, but without wisdom and understanding, accumulated knowledge is not much help.

So, while this book teaches about some things God has given us for our healing, we encourage everyone to ask for wisdom in these matters. We are expecting Him to provide a focused understanding and a release of His compassion for those who are reaching out for His healing hands while reading "Seizing the Kingdom on Healing".

SEIZING THE KINGDOM ON HEALING

CHAPTER 1: God's Medicine Cabinet

Luke 16:8-10 (Paraphrase) *And the lord of his estate praised the unbeliever for what he had done as it was wise.*

The unbelievers are often wiser in relation to their own generation than the believers. Although, Luke 16 is dealing with wisdom concerning money, we often see the unbelievers capturing the wisdom that, we, as believers, are ignorant of in other arenas as well. We have often heard the phrase: "she is so spiritually minded, she is no earthly good". As much as that phrase is distasteful to me, I have to admit that sometimes we can be unwise when it comes to the natural world that God Himself created for our enjoyment. This book will take us back to the Garden of Eden and recapture one of those things that has been credited to the wisdom of the unbeliever, and put it back in its rightful place. That thing is GOD'S BIBLE OILS and that place is the KINGDOM OF GOD. Not only does the bible teach us of these oils, but it states very clearly that there is oil in the house of the WISE!   Proverbs 21:20 *There is precious treasure to be desired and oil in the house of the wise.*

History has proven that in ancient times, Bible oils were an asset to many and brought good health and happiness to those who were fortunate enough to have them in their possession. Today, so many have unknowingly allowed the enemy of our souls to steal this reality from being a blessing in our daily lives.

When we think of the Garden of Eden, what picture do we envision in our minds? Speaking of the terrestrial, we see a vision of purity with trees, fruitful and pleasant to the sight. We behold a flowing river, showcasing abundant fertility and luxuriant vegetation. There, on the landscape of the true Garden of the Lord, we find two people, a man and a woman clothed with garments of light, radiating electricity. They are running barefoot over land that is feeding the electrical system God created within each of them.   A picture of loveliness!   Our God orchestrated it all. Everything He created in the Garden was for maintaining life.

Without electricity, you could not read this book; not because there is not light with which to read, but because your brain wouldn't work. The Lord God made man out of the dust of the earth. That dust has a direct current flowing through it, thus, so does man! Everything we do is controlled and enabled by electrical signals running through our bodies. There is a mass of cells in our heart called the sinoatrial node, or SA node. It's located in the right atrium and it is our body's natural pacemaker. Guess what it takes to set the pace of your blood pumping? You are right: ELECTRICITY. Almost ALL of our cells are capable of generating electricity. But our pulse isn't the only thing that relies on electrical impulses generated by our cells. Later on in this book, we will learn about how we affect the electricity in our bodies when using what God provided: His Bible oils.

Without the trees and plants, Adam and Eve

could not survive. They were for "health maintenance" and now, for us, they are actually for "healing the sick".   Old and New Testament scriptures: Revelation 22:2 *The leaves of the trees are for the healing of the nations.*   Ezekiel 47:12 *Along the bank of the river, on this side and that, will grow all kinds of trees used for food. Their leaves will not wither, and their fruit will be for food, and their leaves shall be for medicine.   Fruit for food, leaves for medicine!* Which sounds better, this prescription or a weight loss pill and an anti-biotic?

Remember Popeye?   Again, the world has displayed wisdom in a simple cartoon show. He ate spinach and became full of strength. Yes, he is a fictional character but the idea is rooted in reality.   It is an example of God's medicine cabinet.

Let's go back to Adam and Eve.   When you envisioned the Garden, did you notice any fragrance? I sensed earth-friendly fragrances. Many, many of them! Some, so delicious that it could make a mouth water while savoring each whiff. Some were pleasant to the smell! What is that soothing, subtle bouquet? Where is that lovely fragrance coming from? How did it benefit Adam and Eve? We are going to discover the answers to these and other questions.

Leaving the Garden now, let's discover what it was about the botanicals, that were so vital to the life of the first earthly parents.

The fruit of the tree for food has no hidden understanding. We all know and understand that trees grow fruit and how good that fruit is for us. What about the leaves of the tree or the leaves of the plants? This has been somewhat allusive to many believers. Oh sure, we all know beet greens are good for us to eat, but what about the leaves of the *patchouli* plant or the *olive* tree leaves? These play an important role in medicinal botany. The oil of these botanicals is the life blood of the plants. The oil is a good analogy to our present understanding that "life is in the blood". The life blood of the plant assists the healing process. For Adam and Eve it was for maintenance AND to aid in healing.

1. Tree Example: The Bible oil *frankincense* is from the Boswellia sacra tree (commonly known as *frankincense* or olibanum-tree) in the Burseraceae family. You probably remember the three wise men brought to honor the baby Jesus! What if I told you one of the wise men was bearing the gift of smooth, flexible, pain-free joints? You might say I'm crazy, but listen to this – An extract of the same tree resin that is used to make *frankincense* has been shown to ease the pain and inflammation of arthritis in as little as seven days according to a study in 2008. **The compound caused no major adverse effects and according to the study authors, is safe for human consumption as well as for those who need it for long-term use:**

Pinterest.com/myhealthjotter/artritis/

Frankincense is regarded the world over as the rarest, most sought after Bible oil in existence. There is an aromatic sap in the Boswellia Tree. Cuts are made in the bark of the tree to harvest the oil. The sap that runs from the cut makes resin tears that dry and harden in the sun.

Differences in climates and soil result in tears of different colors. The lighter–colored tears are said to be of better grade and sell for a higher price. Recent studies have indicated that *frankincense* tree populations are declining. Heavily used trees produce seeds that germinate at only 16% while seeds of trees that had not been used germinate at more than 80%. In addition, burning, grazing, and attacks by long horned beetles have reduced the tree population. Conversion or clearing of *frankincense* woodlands to agriculture is also a threat.

http://en.wikipedia.org/wiki/Frankincense.

This is of great concern and we must use wisdom or lose a very valuable commodity to the world of our health.

2. Plant Example: The Bible oil *patchouli* comes from the *patchouli plant* (Posgostemon cablin). It evokes visions of a beautiful sun and green lawns, but it is far more than that. A less familiar member of the mint family, *patchouli* is distinguished by its' interesting, exotic aroma, but it is far more than that. The health benefits

are far too numerous to list, but includes the treatment of eczema, dermatitis, psoriasis and sores. It provides relief from constipation, and can be used as a temporary antidote or salve against insect bites.

I would wager to say that the majority of the body of Christ does not know this about the Boswellia sacra tree or the *patchouli* plant. Why not? Well, sometimes we are our own worst enemy. Sometimes we get silly with our faith! There is so much in the scriptures concerning God's methods for healing that we could put our faith in, but we have overlooked them, associating so much of the herbs and natural aids with some kind of new age or witchcraft.

Most of the time we've turned to Drs. who use chemicals that poison us, addict us, and even kill us, not to God's life giving substances! You will never hear of someone getting addicted to oil. Just let me say this as we venture into this journey. Biblical remedies and aids for health are all rational and they do not involve incantations or magic rites, nor do they include pharmacy." Biblical therapeutics consisted of washing; the use of oils, balsams, and bandages for wounds and bone fractures; bathing in therapeutic waters, especially in the case of skin diseases; sun rays, medicated drinks, music, etc. Some medical aids for health mentioned by name are *frankincense*, *myrrh*, *cinnamon*, *cassia*, *sandalwood*, *hyssop* and of course, *spikenard*, used on Jesus' feet. The only surgical operations mentioned are circumcision, castration, and embalming.

I know that we all believe in supernatural healing; that God has healed so many of His people instantly! And we love it when He does that, but because of this, we developed a mindset that this is the only way He intends to heal, and it's the only way we want it. This is neither wisdom nor truth. Let us turn to the scripture for understanding God's healing ways. In examining the Greek words for healing, we find several that speak of therapy along with instant, miraculous healing.

1. Therapeuo: This is where our English word

therapeutic comes from, meaning treatment, thus meaning to care for the sick or to restore to health. Therapy! To serve, to give help, take care of another, to cure.

2. Iaomai: Means of physical treatment; a means of healing.

3. therapeia: Medical service, care, healing with the meaning of health.

4. Iasis: Stresses the PROCESS as reaching completion, to heal, unto healing. Luke, the physician used it 15 times. Figuratively, of spiritual and physical healing.

Examples in scripture of therapeutic healings:

1. Ezekiel 30 verse 21 speaks of a man breaking his arm! It says to put the broken arm in a sling so that it may become strong again. Our bodies can heal themselves and the Bible oils assist that healing process. Everything except teeth!

2. Luke 10 verses 33&34 says a Samaritan, as he traveled, came where the (beaten) man was and when he saw him, he took pity on him. He went to him and bandaged his wounds, pouring on oil and wine. Then he

put the man on his own donkey, took him to an inn and took care of him.

When the Lord heals supernaturally, no one has to continue to care for the victim. The Samaritan, of course, was a type of Christ. Wine was used as an anti-septic and since the name of the Bible oil is not listed, we can only surmise as to its kind since the Bible oils all have the capacity to assist in healing our bodies.

3. 2nd Kings 20: 1–7 *In those days, Hezekiah became ill and was at the point of death. The prophet Isaiah, son of Amoz, went to him and said, "This is what the LORD says: Put your house in order, because you are going to die; you will not recover." Hezekiah turned his face to the wall and prayed to the LORD, "Remember, LORD, how I have walked before you faithfully and with wholehearted devotion and have done what is good in your eyes." And Hezekiah wept bitterly. Before Isaiah had left the middle court, the word of the LORD came to him: "Go back and tell*

Hezekiah, the ruler of my people, this is what the LORD, the God of your father David, says: I have heard your prayer and seen your tears; I will heal you. On the third day from now you will go up to the temple of the LORD. I will add fifteen years to your life. And I will deliver you and this city from the hand of the king of Assyria. I will defend this city for my sake and for the sake of my servant David." Then Isaiah said, "Prepare a poultice of figs." They did so and applied it to the boil, and he recovered. A poultice of figs! Who would have guessed? But, do your own research on the oil of figs and you will be amazed at all the health benefits God has given us in this one little fruit.

Just a little side note here: Could you just see Isaiah scratching his head concerning Hezekiah; that when the Lord told him to go to Hezekiah and tell him he was going to die, to get his house in order? Then God tells him to go tell Hezekiah that he is not going to die. I wonder how many of us today could hear God tell us something and then hear that God changed His mind. God changed his mind because of the repentance of the king. Jeremiah 18: 7–11 speaks of the mercy of God toward the repentant heart, changing his mind (thoughts) towards those who humble themselves and turn from whatever may be besetting them. God is spontaneously creative and works all things according to the purpose of His own will. Repenting, forgiving and healing are His will.

4. Psalms 51:7 *Purge me with hyssop and I shall be clean.* One version actually reads: Purge me (from sin with *hyssop*)

I use to read that verse and think, what is this talking about! Purging with *hyssop*? I thought Jesus' blood purged us! Well, little did I understand concerning the oils they used. But David understood. Now, why he didn't go into detail and tell us is fairly obvious. In his day, the people understood he was speaking of the oil of *hyssop* and its ability to help a person overcome addictions. It's obvious why none of the writers went into a great deal of explanation concerning their medicinal practices as their culture understood them. What David was actually asking of the Lord was for some physical help with a physical problem. Along with his repentance, David understood enough to release his faith for deliverance and healing when combining the two. We would call it "a point of contact". Sometimes, a combination of repentance, forgiveness and the oils works miracles.

5. John 19:28-30 When he knew His work was finished, Jesus said he was thirsty. He was offered a sponge soaked in vinegar on a *hyssop* stick. He received it and gave up His spirit. They understood that *hyssop* was also used for emotional balance.

6. Numbers 16:47 We know from this scripture that Aaron stopped the plague with incense and made atonement for the people. If this incense was the same as he was instructed to make in Exodus, the recipe is

given in Exodus 30:34-35. *Take fragrant spices – gum resin, onycha and galbanum – and pure frankincense, all in equal amounts.*

The gum resin mentioned here is called stacte and is simply the sap that drips from the tapping of the wood of the balsam tree, concluded by most that this gum resin is a mixture of Benzoin (*onycha*) and *myrrh*. I can see them placing the oils over the doorpost of their homes and killing the plague. They would place blood on the doorpost. This would attract all the microbes that caused the plague and the oil would kill them. How useful that would be in today's environment. We are constantly being threatened by Ebola outbreaks and pollutants that kill. Today, we have Bible oils useful for stopping plagues. Certainly our children and grandchildren deserve to be protected as they attend school. The anti-septic, anti-viral, and anti-fungal properties in Bible oils of many blends can prevent the air-borne diseases our children tend to bring home with them. We are using this incense recipe only as an example as it was used by Aaron to stop sickness from spreading.

Of the Bible oils mentioned in this verse, we find multiple benefits for the healing of our bodies.

1. _Myrrh_: We know that _myrrh_ was also included in the gifts given to our Lord. It was considered as valuable as the gold brought by the magi. The Ancient Egyptians used it as an antiseptic for an excellent numbing effect. It provides a great deal of immediate relief for pain. _Myrrh_ is a powerful antioxidant: a substance that inhibits oxidation. Topically, myrrh has been used to treat muscular pain. _Myrrh_ can help decrease swelling (inflammation) and kill bacteria. Documented uses and benefits of _myrrh_ are many. To name a few; bronchitis, diabetes, cancer, viral hepatitis, fungal infections, candida, eczema, ringworm, athletes foot, vaginal thrush, tooth and gum conditions, skin conditions, wrinkles, stretch marks, chapped, cracked skin,

diarrhea, dysentery, hyperthyroidism, and ulcers.

2. *Onycha*: Benzoin Bible oil or *onycha* – (styrax benzoin) is extracted from the gum resin. It is a natural anti-inflammatory, anti-septic and a natural wound healer. It is used as a home remedy for bronchitis, rheumatism and skin disorders. Until there was "modern synthetic antiseptics", hospitals used tincture of benzoin. Benzoin is approved by the FDA as a food additive and flavoring agent. Although it may be used as a dietary supplement, it is advised not to use it in this manner with children under six. For therapeutic purposes, use only therapeutic grade Bible oils.

3. *Galbanum*: It has a fresh woody scent. It has detoxifying properties; is good for healing wounds, treats acne, abscesses and boils, is used for depression, is anti-parasitic, promotes the circulation of the blood, inhibits fungal or microbial growth in cuts, etc., a decongestant, anti-

spasmodic, natural relaxant and diminishes scars.

4. _Frankincense_: We have already mentioned arthritis is helped by using this oil. _Frankincense_ has antiseptic, disinfectant, digestive, diuretic, and sedative properties. We can understand why Aaron and other Bible figures would use it as fumes or smoke. The antiseptic and disinfectant qualities eliminated the germs in the space they were using when the smoke filtered out. It helps our skin, menstruation, anti-aging, and uterine health. People boast of less stress and anxiety using a blend of oils, when _frankincense_ and _myrrh_ are the main ingredients.

There are a few scriptural references to therapy; 36 of the 39 books of the Old Testament and 10 of the 27 books of the New Testament mention Bible oils or the plants that produce them. These are the medicines provided by our Lord! I think we can conclude that the oils in the leaves of the trees and the plants were indeed in God's medicine cabinet.

SEIZING THE KINGDOM ON HEALING

CHAPTER 2 – The Help of Science

Most laymen know there is a real problem with modern medicine and many prefer not to use it. We are so thankful for the many, many times that modern medicine has saved a life through surgery or emergency treatment. It definitely has its place, but all too often it steps beyond what most of us would call safe and sound treatment. Prescription, or over the counter drugs just temporarily relieve symptom. Today, we can thank modern science for showing pharmaceuticals up for the safe boundaries they has crossed. Science has discovered many principles of wholesome health, but these discoveries originated with God who designed and created the miracles in the human body. Our Creator God, whom we know as the Great physician, knows everything about us. He has provided medicine for healing and maintaining good health, not just temporarily covering symptoms in the body. We are thankful today that scientists have discovered what God set in motion is true. Three chemicals in the Bible oils do what modern medicine cannot. The use of modern medicine cannot go behind the blood brain barrier. If we cannot get past this barrier with pharmaceuticals, then we cannot get healed with over the counter or prescription medication. We can stop having the symptoms of a specific illness, but its' effects are destroying something somewhere else in the body, thus, would it not be safe to say "modern medicines do not heal"? According to science, there is a reason. The molecules of pharmaceutical drugs are very large. Large molecules cannot penetrate the blood brain barrier where healing takes place. Here is the wisdom of God: He made the molecules in the Bible oils very tiny. Tiny molecules _do_ penetrate the blood brain barrier and heal, with no adverse effects. Once the oils go past this barrier, they are able to do three things that assist in healing because of their chemical components working in unison to restore our bodies back to its natural state of balance and health.

Working then, at the most basic, fundamental

level of the cells, these three chemicals are:

1. Phenolpropanoids: Cleanses the receptor site on the surface of the cells. Think of it as cleaning your windows. This chemical is the spray coming from your bottle and the rag in your hand. It lands on the window and you wipe it clean. This chemical lands on your cells and cleanses the receptor sites clean.

2. Sesquitterpenes: Deprograms   bad information in the cell at the subcellular level by facilitating oxygen transfer. Think of this chemical as kicking a thief out of your house.

3. Monoterpenes: Reprograms the cells with correct information at both the subcellular and intracellular levels.   Think of it as changing a misspelled word in a document.

Even inherited conditions can be reprogrammed in the DNA of the cells by the assistance of Bible oils. They will help restore the body back to its natural state of balance. Simply put, the oils rewrite, miswritten DNA. You are not at the mercy of the DNA in your cells. We can thank the world of science for giving us this knowledge. Because the DNA of the cells can be re-written, the Bible oils are capable of helping the emotions as well. Our brains are like libraries. They catalogue every thought we have somewhere in the body. When a person has an emotional experience, good or bad, it deposits itself within our cells. When it is a bad experience, it shows up as a sickness in one of many places, from the head to the toes. Because of the properties of the cells, they can assist in the healing process by cleansing the cells and thereby release emotions connected with the bad experience. Truly, you are not at the mercy of DNA.

The oils have electrical properties. Since we were created from the dust of the ground, it is a logical conclusion that we also contain the same electrical current as the ground. As we stated earlier, this current is a direct current. It wasn't wisdom to put alternating current in homes as it goes against the flow of the blood. In alternating current, the flow of electric charge periodically reverses direction. In direct current, the flow of electric charge is only in one direction. Have you ever had your radio on and driven under the wires over the road? If you have, you heard the radio go into static mode. This is because the wires above you are alternating current and your radio is direct current. This is what AC does to our blood flow. We could use some help in the flow of our blood. In one study two men measured 66MHz. One held a cup of coffee (without drinking any) and his frequency dropped to 58MHz in 3 seconds. Within 21 seconds after inhaling the aroma of the bible oils his frequency had returned to 66 MHZ. A second male test subject drank a sip of coffee. His MHz also dropped... to 52 MHZ. He did not use the oils and it took him 3 days for his frequency to return to the initial 66 MHZ. Oils are frequency-specific subtle energy in the form of vibrational medicine and can change dysfunctional energy patterns — Richard Gerber MD, author of "Vibrational Medicine".

In 1992, it was discovered that oils have a bio-electrical frequency. Their frequencies are the highest of all known substances. One of their most important roles is to lift our bodily frequencies to levels where disease cannot exist. A person's health can be determined by the frequency of the person's body. Frequencies are also affected by thought... Thus the advice to <u>pray</u> when using the Bible oils! Sometimes repentance and prayer are necessary. Negative thoughts lower the frequency of the oils and positive thoughts raise the frequency. It stands to reason then, that praying while you use the oils would make the greatest difference. The energetic vibration of the plant unites with the harmony of our "electric" bodies. When you are inhaling a pure Bible oil, you are connecting to the very Life Power of the plant.

When God said, *"Let the earth bring forth vegetation, the herb yielding seed after its kind"*, our plants and trees became a direct creation of His word. Properly applied in a prayerful way, they possess a Divine understanding. They know how to do what is beneficial and how to avoid doing anything that will bring harm. Once again, science confirms this fact.

Let's take a look at what happens, for instance, when we take an anti-biotic. First, consider the source of antibiotics!

Antibiotics work in one of a few ways: by either interfering with the bacteria's ability to repair its damaged DNA, by stopping the bacteria's ability to make what it needs to grow new cells, or by weakening the bacteria's cell wall until it bursts. That is all well and good, however, taking antibiotics comes with some risk. Some antibiotics are associated with nasty side effects; while they are designed to kill the infection-causing bacteria in your body, they also cause problems when they kill the good bacteria living inside you. They lie to our bodies. They are not created from truth. Antibiotics may cause vaginal infections (what we commonly call yeast infections), as well as upset stomach and diarrhea, among other problems. Antibiotics are designed to kill a specific type of bacteria and the body's own built in defense mechanism can build up such a resistance to the antibiotic that it will become ineffective, requiring a much more potent antibiotic. There will come a day when we reach the end of the potency required for diseases and what will happen then? Antibiotics will be a thing of the past.

Source: http://www.cdc.gov/drugresistance/threat-report-2013. I say, "Good". It could not happen too soon. Let's get back to what God has given us that *does not lie* to our bodies; that *does not* have any bad side effects, and that destroys only the bad bacteria: God's Bible Oils! His oils speak the truth to our bodies because they are born of the truth.

Most of the Bible oils have properties as an antiseptic, disinfectant, astringent, carminative (relieves flatulence), cicatrizing (healing of a wound otherwise than by first intention), cytophlactic, (protects the cells of an organism) digestive, diuretic, emenagogue, expectorant, sedative, tonic uterine and vulnerary substance (assists in the healing of wounds). These properties allow the Bible oils to assist healing as God intended, not using abrasive treatment methods with so many side effects and addictive killing substances.

Decades of clinical experience by doctors in France suggests that Bible oils frequently heal both acute and chronic infections without the damaging, and often long-lasting effect on bowel flora that comes from the use of antibiotics. But, with or without any evidence, experiential or otherwise, our evidence is what God says about it. We aren't saying Bible oils heal. God's word says it.

Again, Ezekiel 47:12 *Fruit trees of all kinds will grow on both banks of the river. Their leaves will not wither, nor will their fruit fail. Every month they will bear fruit, because the water from the sanctuary flows to them. Their fruit will serve for food and their <u>leaves for healing</u>* (medicine).

Threat Report 2013: This report states, Antibiotic resistance threats in the United States in 2013 gives a first-ever snapshot of the burden and threats posed by the antibiotic-resistant germs having the most impact on human health. Each year in the United States, at least 2 million people become infected with bacteria that are resistant to antibiotics and at least 23,000 people die each year as a direct result of these infections. Many more people die from other conditions that were complicated by an antibiotic-resistant infection.

Antibiotic-resistant infections can happen anywhere. Data show that most happen in the general community; however, most deaths related to antibiotic resistance happen in healthcare settings such as hospitals and nursing homes."

Source:

http://www.cdc.gov/drugresistance/threat-report-2013

It has been reported that thyme and cinnamon are particularly good anti-bacterial agents when combating infections of many kinds. Not only are Bible oils a less expensive treatment but the less we use antibiotics the better. God's class of "antibiotics" in NON-toxic forms are much more effective, far less expensive and much more flexible than Big Pharma could ever hope to create. There has been no recognition by the medical profession as a whole of the importance of the "QUALITY" of the therapeutic value of God's kind of medicine. However, why would we listen to what they say as their own research reports are always contradicting each other? One day, one thing is good for you and the next it is harmful. They seem to be very confused!

Clinical studies are currently underway in Europe, Australia, Japan, India, the United States, and Canada. Many of these studies describe the remarkable properties that assist healing, using the various oils.

Many conventional drug studies are funded by the pharmaceutical industry itself. There is not motivation for these companies to fund research on natural plant substances because they cannot easily be patented, limiting potential for profit. They also have difficulty testing as the times for harvesting plants and trees will make a difference in their findings. Thus, finding funding for Bible oil studies can be challenging. The research that has been done on Bible oils show positive effects for a variety of health concerns including infections, pain, anxiety, depression, tumors, premenstrual syndrome, nausea, and many others. However, what difference does this make to us as believers; we have God's word on it!

Another discovery we want to take a look at is the ORAC value of the oils. ORAC stands for Oxygen Radical Absorption Capacity. We can actually thank the US Department of Agriculture for establishing the ORAC values on our foods, juices and oils for this research. This value measures anti-oxidant capacities. An anti-oxidant is a substance that inhibits oxidation. If you slice an apple and don't eat it, it will turn brown. Leave fish on the cupboard and what happens? It becomes rancid! A cut anywhere on your body can become inflamed. This will happen naturally because of oxidation. Antioxidants are crucial to your health. When a cell doesn't get enough antioxidants, it becomes damaged and turns into a free radical looking for another cell to make up what it has lost. Antioxidants destroy free radicals; thus retards the aging process and prevents diseases. Free radicals are a reactive atom or group of atoms that has one or more unpaired electrons; especially: one that is produced in the body by natural biological processes or introduced from an outside source (hair spray, tobacco smoke, toxins, or pollutants) and that can damage cells, proteins, and DNA by altering their chemical structure.

Just to give you an example of the power of the Bible oils: Let's compare cauliflower to clove, (the highest scoring Bible oil). Cauliflower's score is 136 and the oil of clove scores 290,283. Now, admittedly scores vary depending on which charts you look at, but they all have these wide spread scores between cauliflower and clove. Bible oils scored as the highest source we have for destroying free radicals. Everything else pales in comparison. The USDA published the ORAC value scores in 2010 and then two years later retracted their findings. This is the type of thing that makes you go hmmmm! Perhaps they didn't like that the oils rated so high???

We could go on and on with evidence that man has discovered, but we think this suffices for now. Man's continual searching will only support what God has already told us whether we understand it scientifically or not.

CHAPTER 3 – "Salt 'N Oil"

SALT:

Speaking of God's people, the scripture says: "My people are destroyed for lack of knowledge". It is unhealthy for us when we do not understand what is in the food we eat as so much of it is full of disease causing microbes. It is bad enough what the growers use for fertilizer and the things that are added to it before it even reaches us, but we are addressing here, in this chapter, the natural fungi that is already in the food. The above scripture goes on to say this: "because they rejected knowledge".

This is our opportunity to receive knowledge that will bring us life and healthy habits with our meal preparations.

We cannot depend upon the government to correctly regulate our food. This has become so much more evident during this past decade. The introduction of genetically modified organisms to the blind eye given to carcenegentics, and the obvious feelings of the FDA to keep our drugs and food within a safe range, has triggered a movement toward the natural; the life given elements coming unaltered from our earth.

We have significant evidence today that we are actually killing ourselves by what we eat and how we eat it.   Our food, like pharmaceutical medications, is like a long term time bomb. No, we don't see the evidence immediately, but over years and sometimes days, we feel the adverse effects of what we put in our bodies.

Wouldn't you like to chomp down on that New York steak and know that the dangerous fungi have been removed? But, that fungi is in the blood that is still in the meat you eat. There was a reason the Apostle Paul said to refrain from meat strangled with blood. An animal that was snared and killed by strangling (choking), still had blood in it. It was against the law to strangle an animal (cruelty) in the Old Testament. Perhaps, cruelty is part of the reason behind Paul's statement, however everyone knows whatever method is used to kill livestock blood is still in the meat. Just let it sit out for a few moments, just let it sit a few moments after it is cooked. What happens? Blood runs out! So, if you eat that piece of meat without cleaning it first, you are eating the blood that is full of microbes (dangerous fungi). We clean our vegetables, but for the most part, we have never learned to clean our red meats and poultry. We are going to learn how, now.

1. Wash the meat or fowl thoroughly to remove any visible blood.
2. Immerse the meat in water.
3. Let it sit for an hour.
4. Rinse and drain the water.
5. Salt the meat thoroughly -- top, bottom and sides -- with coarse "REAL" sea salt. Do not put so much salt on the meat that blood cannot drain out, but keep the meat

damp enough so salt sticks to it; not so wet that the salt dissolves easily.

6. Place it in the refrigerator for an hour.
7. Rinse with water and it is ready to cook.

This salt process removes all the mycotoxins (fungi) from your meats. It will only change the color of the meat, not the flavor and now you have meat for your meal that you know is not going to be disastrous for your health in the long run.

It is also important to mention the fat of the meat. Fungi hides in the fat as well as the blood. Again, wisdom says, "do not eat any of the fat"! The Real salt we mentioned is a brand of sea salt we recommend because it has the highest pH factor of any sea salt. This salt contains antifungals that are excellent fungi fighters, whereas the normal table salt contains things that are not good for us; things that can actually make us sick over a period of time. Most common table salt is made up of chemicals that pollute our bodies and wreak havoc on our health. Healthy natural sea salts contain no toxins and over 84 minerals and elements necessary for your optimal health. Regular table salt is actually 97.5% sodium chloride and 2.5% chemicals such as moisture absorbents, and iodine. Because the salt is dried at over 1,200 degrees Fahrenheit, the excessive heat alters the natural chemical structure of the salt, destroying salt's natural nutrient. The body itself recognizes normal table salt as something completely foreign. As a food, typical table salt is absolutely useless, and can potentially act as a destructive poison. In order for the body to metabolize table salt crystals, it must sacrifice tremendous amounts of energy. Inorganic sodium chloride upsets the fluid balance and constantly overburdens your elimination systems. Aluminum hydroxide is often added to improve the ability of table salt to pour. Aluminum is a light alloy that deposits into your brain – a potential cause of Alzheimer's disease. This is why your Dr. tells you not to eat salt. It is hard on you. But not Real Salt. Salt is not bad for you; it is altered table salt that is bad for you. This is confirmed in the scriptures (authoritative writings).

Sea salt is rapidly becoming more popular, as more and more people are learning about all the health benefits that the salt has to offer. The salt is obtained naturally from the sea, and does not go through any processing that alters it, retaining the natural minerals.

Information of the health benefits of sea salt have been made available to us by Ready Nutrition, originally published September 15th, 2001 as below.

Strong Immune System – Sea salt naturally helps you to build up a strong immune system so that you can fight off the cold virus, the fever and flu, allergies and other autoimmune disorders.

Alkalizing – Sea salt is alkalizing to the body, as it has not been exposed to high heat and stripped of its minerals, nor does it have any harmful man-made ingredients added to it. Thus it can help you to prevent and reverse high levels of acids in the body, which in turn eliminates the risks for serious and life-threatening diseases.

Weight Loss – Believe it or not, but sea salt can also help you in weight loss. It helps the body to create digestive juices so that the foods you eat are digested faster, and it helps to prevent buildup in the digestive tract, which eventually can lead to constipation and weight gain.

Skin Conditions – A sea salt bath can help to relieve dry and itchy skin as well as serious conditions such as eczema and psoriasis. The bath naturally opens up the pores, improves circulation in the skin and hydrates the tissues so that your skin can heal.

Asthma – Sea salt is effective in reducing inflammation in the respiratory system. Thus the production of phlegm is slowed down so that you can breathe easier again. Some say that sprinkling sea salt on the tongue after drinking a glass of water is just as effective as using an inhaler. But the great thing about sea salt is that it has no side effects when taken in moderation.

Heart Health – When sea salt is taken with water it can help to reduce high cholesterol levels, high blood pressure and help to regulate an irregular heartbeat. Thus sea salt can help to prevent atherosclerosis, heart attacks and strokes.

Diabetes – Sea salt can help to reduce the need of insulin by helping to maintain proper sugar levels in the body. Thus the salt is an essential part of the diet if you are diabetic, or at risk for the disease.

Osteoporosis – Just over 1/4 of the amount of salt that is in the body is stored in the bones, where it helps to keep them strong. When the body lacks salt and water it begins to draw the sodium from the bones, which then eventually can lead to osteoporosis. Thus by drinking plenty of water and consuming salt in moderation you can prevent osteoporosis.

Muscle Spasms – Potassium is essential for helping the muscles to function properly. Sea salt not only contains small amounts of potassium, but it also helps the body to absorb it better from other foods. Thus it is effective in helping to prevent muscle pains, spasms and cramps.

Depression – Sea salt also has shown to be effective in treating various types of depression. The salt helps to preserve two essential hormones in the body that help you to better deal with stress. These hormones are serotonin and melatonin, which help you to feel good, and relax and sleep better at night.

What the Supreme Authority has to say about salt:

There are some Hebrew idioms in the Bible concerning salt and it would seem fitting to mention a couple here, simply for a fun educational moment. An idiom is a "saying" that foreigners cannot understand without being trained and is often taken literally and therefore misunderstood. This is because when we use an idiom we say one thing, but we mean another.

1. Genesis 19:26 *And she became a pillar of salt. Idiom for "she became petrified with fear and died".*

2. Matthew 5:13 *Salt of the earth. Idiom for "good conduct".*

3. Mark 9:50 *Have salt in yourselves. Idiom for "have good manners".*

Salt is an emblem of the covenant between God and His people. This quite possibly is because natural salt itself is purifying, perpetuating, and has antiseptic properties. Every meal offering in the Old Testament was to contain salt.

Leviticus 2:13 *Season all your grain offerings with salt to remind you of God's eternal covenant. Never forget to add salt to your grain offerings.*

The Israelites offered meal (cereals) or vegetables in addition to the animals. Leviticus Chapter 2 mentions four kinds of cereal offerings and gives cooking instructions for each. The sinner could offer dough from wheat flour baked in an oven, cooked on a griddle, fried in a pan, or roasted to make bread (as in the offering of the first fruits). All meal offerings were made with salt and oil, and no honey and leaven were to be used (salt and oil preserved while honey and leaven would spoil). The worshipper was also to bring a portion of incense (*frankincense*).

The meal offerings were brought to one of the priests, who took it to the altar and cast a "memorial portion" on the fire and he also did this with the incense. He ate what remained unless he was bringing the meal offering for himself, then he would burn the whole thing.

If God thought salt was bad for us, He definitely would have instructed the priests NOT to eat of the meal offerings. Yes? Yes!

2nd Kings 2:19-21 *Then the men of the city said to Elisha, "Behold now, the situation of this city is pleasant, as my lord sees; but the water is bad and the land is unfruitful." He said, "Bring me a new jar, and put salt in it." So they brought it to him. He went out to the spring of water and threw salt in it and said, Thus says the LORD, "I have purified these waters; there shall not be from thence any more death or unfruitfulness any longer".*

That wasn't a miracle. The salt cleaned the water.

However, when God instructed a Prophet to "throw salt on the ground", it's meaning was to keep the area from being productive again; even full cities were destroyed in such a manner to never again be rebuilt permanently: Samaria,

Ninevah, Ashkelon, Edom, Tyre, Chorazin, and Bethsaida. Salt would "kill" the ground.

Mark 9:50 *Salt is good for seasoning. But if it loses its flavor, how do you make it salty again? You must have the qualities of salt among yourselves and live in peace with each other.*

We understand this is speaking about believers, but the comparison is very plain. We are being compared to the qualities of salt. Typical table salt has lost its savor and cannot be of any more benefit to us. The qualities of a true Bible salt is a great comparison to believers. QUALITIES of a good salt: In short: Sodium chloride, an abundant mineral in salt. Sodium chloride inhalation can remove certain bacteria in body secretions. It is a preservative. A little salt sets the flavor in food. Salt has healing properties. It kills most germs on contact. It burns when it hits a raw spot, but is very effective in cleansing a wound so it can heal. "Don't rub salt in my wounds", is an idiom we use in America that is often said when a person doesn't like having good advice given to him/her.

So have a little salt every day! "Real salt", that is!

We recommend you use a 5% solution (5 parts cider/95 parts water) of organic apple cider vinegar to clean your fruits and vegetables. For years our parents used baking soda for upset stomachs or heart burn. We had less cancer then! The pH of baking soda (sodium bicarbonate $NaHCO_3$ is pH 8.2.) It's important to keep your pH level balanced. This is better for your health and is quite inexpensive. We recommend using ½ c. water and ¼ teaspoon baking soda upon rising and again when retiring for the night. You can buy pH test strips at most health food stores and some grocery stores. You will be so happy to see your pH level go to a balanced state (alkaline–7.3) using the soda regularly.

<u>OIL:</u>

What kind and why? The *olive* was one of the most valuable trees to the ancient Hebrews. It is first mentioned in Scripture when the dove returned to Noah's ark carrying an *olive* branch in its beak (Genesis 8:11). Since that time, the *olive* branch has been a symbol of "peace" to the world, and we often hear the expression, "extending an *olive* branch" to another person as a desire for peace.

The Hebrew word for "*olive* tree" is *es shemen,* which literally means 'tree of oil." It is from a primitive root meaning "to shine." It means "richness, anointing, fat, and fruitful, oil, ointment, olive." It is related to the word *shemesh,* "to be brilliant," and which also is the Hebrew word for the "sun," that brightly shining orb in the sky.

Another Hebrew word for "*olive*" is *zayith,* meaning "an *olive*," as "yielding illuminating oil." It's related to the word *ziv,* meaning "to be prominent," "brightness."

Olive oil was used as a medicine and as staple in the diets of the Hebrew people.

Leviticus 6:14–15 The Grain Offering: *"Now this is the law of the grain offering: the sons of Aaron shall present it before the LORD in front of the altar. Then one of them shall lift up from* it a handful of the fine flour of the grain offering, with its oil and all the incense that is on the grain offering, and he shall offer it up in smoke on the altar, a soothing aroma, as its memorial offering to the LORD."

Leviticus 2:1 *When anyone brings a grain/cereal offering to the LORD, their offering is to be of the finest flour. They are to pour olive oil on it!*

There was a good reason that *olive* oil was to be used on All the grains; it kills mycotoxins. *Olive* oil is highly antifungal. It protects our bodies from disease and illness. *Olive* leaf extract powdered tea kills fungi.

A few years ago, I picked up a spore in a dusty old building. The Drs. treated me for a bacteria with the usual antibiotic, etc., all to no avail. It left me weak; I coughed so hard I fractured a rib and for eleven months I was forced to spend my nights in a sitting position just to breathe. My friend told me to get a corn cob pipe and put some crushed *olive* leaves from his tree in it and smoke it. Through the therapy of that corn cob pipe, filled with *olive* leaves, my lungs cleared up because the real problem was a fungus, not a bacteria.

When lepers were cleansed, a special sacrifice was made together with "fine flour mixed with *olive* oil as a grain offering, and one log of oil" (Leviticus14:10). A "log" was a little over a half a quart. At the cleansing ceremony, a lamb was slain as a trespass offering, and a log of oil, both waved as a wave offering before the Lord. The priest would pour some of the oil into his own left hand, then dip his right finger into the oil in his left hand, and sprinkle the oil seven times before the Lord, and of the rest of the oil in his left hand he would put some on the tip (lobe) of the right ear of the leper being cleansed, and on the thumb of his right hand, and on the big toe of his right foot. (Lev. 14-13-18). The rest of the oil would be put on his head. The brain stem runs to the tip of the ear lobe and when oil is placed on it, its benefits run extremely fast to the brain... How fast? Faster than a speeding locomotive. Look everyone, it's Superoil! It's Extra Virgin *Olive* Oil...

1. The *olive* oil produced from the first hour of cold-pressing (low temperatures) whole olives, is called Extra Virgin. This oil retains all of its flavor, aroma, and nutritional value.
2. The *olive* oil produced after the first hour is called Virgin and after an allotted time, what is left to press is called *Olive* Oil.

Heat destroys the benefits of Extra Virgin so we recommend you use the less expensive *olive* oil for cooking. Unsparingly, use the Extra Virgin on your salads and anything else you would enjoy it on. It is full of so much value for your health. Kill those microbes in pasta...douse it well. (No pun intended) Sprinkle it over veggies. There are some really good Extra Virgin oils on the market. Some have a lively *olive* flavor with a mild peppery finish that is absolutely delicious, even over meats.

Because there is so much marketing fraud on good extra virgin *olive* oil, I thought our readers

would appreciate knowing the following. In September 2012, Consumer Reports published its results from testing 23 *olive* oils from Italy, Spain and California, and only 9 passed the test as actually being extra virgin *olive* oil, as claimed on the label. Two that failed? Bertolli and Goya. Two that passed? McEvoy Ranch and Trader Joe's California Estate. – See more at: http://www.
phoenixhelix.com/2013/03/04/
would-the-real-olive-oil-please-stand
up/#sthash.pBzzgl2v.dpuf.

It can also be purchased on Amazon.com.

CHAPTER 4: Priesthood of the Believer

In this chapter we will endeavor to answer four questions: Where are the priests today? Where is God's temple and altar today? Who were the healers in the bible? What did they use for medicine?

The first mention of a priest in the bible was Melchezidek. Aaron, born a Levite, was High Priest of the Old Covenant.

Aaron's mother, Jochebed, the Egyptian-born daughter of Levi, married her nephew Amram son of Kohath, and gave birth to three children: Miriam, the eldest; Aaron; and Moses, the youngest, who was born when Aaron was three years old. Part of the Law (Torah) that Moses received from God at Sinai granted Aaron the priesthood for himself and his male descendants, and as such, he became the first high priest of the Israeli nation.

Exodus 28:1 *Then bring near to you and Aaron and his sons with him, from among the peoples* of Israel, to serve me as priests—Aaron and Aaron's sons, Nadab and Abihu, Eleazar and Ithamar.

The high priests were not only the religious leaders of their day, but they were also considered the Supreme leaders over all priests with duties designated specifically to them.

Exodus 29: 7 (Speaking of Aaron) *You shall take the anointing oil and pour it on his head and anoint him.*

Anointing the head of the high priests with oil was full of significance. From a cultural viewpoint, we have lost most of the significance of the anointing with oil as we have viewed it as merely a type of the Holy Spirit, which it is. However, anoint means an ointment. The ointment used was not merely some olive oil dabbed on the head. The Bible records often, that a great amount of oil was used in consecrations and healings as well as burials. We now understand that it is not just the oil itself that is a type, but the properties of the oils are also significant in meaning when used as an ointment when we pray for healing.

One of the principle duties of Aaron and his sons was to offer sacrifices.

Leviticus 16:14-15 The most important duty of the high priest was to conduct the service on the Day of Atonement, the tenth day of the seventh month of every year. Only he was allowed to enter the Most Holy Place behind the veil to stand before God. Having made a sacrifice for himself and for the people, he then brought the blood into the Holy of Holies and sprinkled it on the mercy seat, God's throne. He did this to make atonement for himself and the people for all their sins committed during the year just ended (Exodus 30:10).

Did you ever wonder with all that blood poured on the altar, how they kept from getting sick; plagued with diseases? It was the properties in the oils they used in their service. They were anti-bacterial, anti-fungal, anti-viral, etc. in nature.

Numbers 18: 5 Another duty of the high priests was the responsibility for the ministering around the sanctuary and the altar. God had set Aaron and his sons apart, anointing them for service. Anointing is used many places in the Bible to set people apart for service. Both these things are important to remember as we consider where God's "sanctuary and altar are today" and also knowing that the oil is a type of the Holy Spirit, as we consider "where the priests are today".

2nd Chronicles 29:34 After the call of Aaron as a high priest, God called several others taken from the tribe of Levi. His purpose in doing this was so that the high priests would not be overworked. These Levites were considered assistants to the high priests.

Numbers 3:5-9 *The Lord said to Moses, "Bring the tribe of Levi and present them to Aaron the high priest to assist him. They are to perform duties for him and for the whole community at the tent of meeting by doing the work of the tabernacle. They are to take care of the furnishings of the tent of meeting, fulfilling the obligations of the Israelites by doing the work of the tabernacle. Give the Levites to Aaron and his sons; they are the Israelites who are given to be given wholly to him".*

These Levites also taught the written Law and administered justice. They were responsible for assembling, dismantling, and transporting the Tabernacle.

According to Numbers 8:24–25 these Levitical priests served for 25 years, from age 25 to age 50.

Other than the family of Aaron, there were only three other family lines in the tribe of Levi (Numbers chapter 4): the Kohathites, who maintained the furniture, vessels and veil of the Tabernacle; the Gershonites, who maintained the coverings, hangings and doors of the Tabernacle; the Merarites, who maintained the supports, including the planks bars and cords, of the Tabernacle.

Initially, God had selected the entire nation of Israel to be his priests, according to Exodus 19:5,6; however, after the nation proved to be inadequate as priests, Exodus 32:7-10, the Levites who supported Moses in Exodus chs. 26 and 28 were selected as God's priests. We find this in the scripture we already quoted: Numbers 3:5–9.

The Old Testament Priesthood became extinct at the destruction of Jerusalem.

This brings us to "where are the priests today"?

A NEW ORDER IS INTRODUCED:

This new order:

1. <u>Would be superior to the Levitical priesthood:</u>
   Hebrews 7:4–7
   Now observe and consider how great this man was to whom even Abraham the patriarch gave a tenth of the heap of the spoils. And it is true that those descendants of Levi who are charged with the priestly office are commanded in the Law to take tithes from the people, which means their brethren, though they came out of the loins of Abraham. But this person who has not their Levitical ancestry received tithes from Abraham himself, and blessed him who possessed the promises of God.

Yet it is beyond all contradiction that it is the lesser person who is blessed by the greater one.

2. <u>Would not depend upon ancestry</u>:
   Hebrews 7:14
   For it is obvious that our Lord sprang from the tribe of Judah, and Moses mentioned nothing about priests in connection with that tribe.

3. <u>Would have a priest who is both King and Priest</u>:
   Zechariah 6:12–13
   And speak unto Joshua saying, Thus says the Lord of Hosts (Captain of the army) Behold the Man (the Messiah) whose name is the Branch, for He shall grow up in His place, and He shall build the true temple of the Lord. Yes, there is a temple being built, but it is He Who shall build the true temple of the Lord and He shall bear the honor and the glory, and shall sit and rule upon His throne. And He shall be a priest upon

His thrown, and the counsel of peace shall be between the two offices, Priest and King. See also: (John 1:14; 17:5; Hebrews, 2:9)

4. <u>Would not be from the loins of Abraham, Father of the Jewish nation</u>:

   Hebrews 7:3-4 *Without father, without mother, without descent, having neither beginning of days, nor end of life; but made like unto the Son of God; abiding a priest continually. Now consider how great this man was, unto whom even the patriarch Abraham gave the tenth of the spoils.*

Here we come back, full circle to the first mention of a priest in the scriptures. He is the beginning and the consummation.

Why was it necessary for a new order? Perfection did not come through the Old Testament priesthood.

Hebrews 7:11 *If therefore perfection were by the Levitical priesthood, for under it, the people received the LAW what further need would there have been that another priest should rise after the order of Melchezidek and not be called after the order and rank of Aaron.*

The LAW could not redeem anyone. It was a glory; it was of God, but no one wanted to keep it and when they were unwilling to live by it, it caused death.

Hebrews 7:19 *For there is verily a disannulling of the commandment going before for the ineffectiveness thereof. For the law made nothing perfect, but the bringing in of a better hope (covenant) did; by which we draw nigh unto God.*

So, we see the Old Covenant was the letter that kills whereas the New Covenant is the Spirit that gives life.

Jesus, being our High Priest has now mediated a better covenant whereby He is known as the chief Cornerstone.

1st Peter 2:6 *Behold, I lay in Zion a chief Cornerstone.*

1st Peter 2:3-5: *Since you have tasted the goodness and kindness of the Lord, Come to*

Him; that Living Stone which men tried and threw away, but which is chosen and precious in God's sight. COME and as living stones yourselves be built into a spiritual house to be a holy priesthood, to offer up spiritual sacrifices that are acceptable and well-pleasing to God through Jesus Christ.

1st Peter 2:9 *You are a chosen generation, a royal priesthood, an holy nation, a people of God's own possession, that you may proclaim the excellencies of Him who has called you out of darkness into His marvelous light.*

Answer # 1 Where are the priests today? All who have come to know Jesus as the Lord are priests according to the scriptures.

Question #2 Where are the temple and the altar thereof today?

Everything changed at the destruction of Jerusalem.

There was of necessity a change of the LAW and

a change of the priesthood. But what happened to the temple and the altar of sacrifice?

This is a prophecy Jesus gave to a disciple concerning the temple.

Mark 13:1-2 *And as he went out of the temple, one of his disciples said unto him, Master, notice the quality of stones and what buildings are here! Jesus answered him saying, "You see these great buildings? There will not be left here one stone upon another that will not be loosened and torn down".*

On another occasion Jesus foretold the destruction of Jerusalem. It was when he entered the city and the people laid their clothes on the ground before him, this being the custom to give honor to someone of great importance.

Luke 19:36-46 *Then the crowds spread out their robes along the road ahead of him, and as they reached the place where the road started down from the Mount of Olives, the whole procession began to shout and sing as they walked along, praising God for all the wonderful miracles Jesus did. God has given us a King, they exulted. Long live the King! Let all heaven rejoice! Glory to God in the highest heavens!!!!!!*

But some of the Pharisees among the crowd said, 'Sir, rebuke your followers for saying things like that!' Jesus replied, 'If they keep quiet, the stones along the road will burst into cheers!' But as they came closer to Jerusalem and he saw the city ahead, he began to cry. "Eternal peace was within your reach and you turned it down,' he wept, 'and now it is too late. Your enemies will pile up earth against your walls and encircle you and close in on you, and crush you to the ground, and your children within you; <u>your enemies will not leave one stone upon another</u> for you have rejected the opportunity God offered you." Then he entered the Temple and began to drive out the merchants from their stalls, saying to them, "The Scriptures declare, My Temple is a place of prayer; but you have turned it into a den of thieves".

Although Jesus understood that his heavenly Father was merciful, he also understood the heart of the vast majority of the religious at that time; their corrupt leadership and that they would not repent of their evil ways. This is one of the reasons he wept over Jerusalem as he foretold its destruction and the complete annihilation of the temple.

Three things take place now that complete the setting of the changes made to the priesthood, the law and the temple with the altar.

1. Jesus is acknowledged as the Son of God:

   Matthew 27:54 *And when Jesus had cried with a loud voice, he said, "Father, into thy hands I commend my spirit": and having said thus, he gave up the ghost. Now when the centurion saw what was done, he glorified God, saying, "Certainly this man was the Son of God".*

2. The relationship with God changed:

Mark 15: 37-38 *And Jesus cried with a loud voice, and breathed out his life... And the veil (curtain) of the temple was torn in half from the top to the bottom. At that moment, the relationship between God and humanity was forever changed. Now, the way is forever open for all humanity to have direct fellowship with God our Father.*

3. The place of worship changed:

John.4:19-23 *The Samaritan woman said to Jesus: "Sir, I perceive that thou art a Prophet. Our forefathers worshipped on this mountain, but you Jews say we must worship at Jerusalem"! Jesus replied, "Woman, a time is coming when neither in this mountain, nor in Jerusalem, shall you worship the Father."*

Now there is no difference between the Jew and the Greek: for the same Lord over all is rich unto all that call upon him in faith.

In Christ, those who were afar off from the commonwealth of Israel are now able to have communion with God with no requirement of going through a natural man. Any who worship can now be anywhere at any time, presenting their own petitions and know that He will hear.

So, the old temple in Jerusalem was destroyed; Jerusalem itself was destroyed. The prophecies all came true. There was so much gold lining the walls of the temple that when the Romans fulfilled the prophecies of Jesus Christ, by destroying it in 70 AD, the fire actually melted the gold and they turned over every stone trying to retrieve it. It caused the land to look as if there was never a city there.

Do you still desire to be under the law? Do you still desire a natural man for a priest?

Galatians 4:21-31 *Tell me, you who are bent on being under the law, do ye not hear the law? For it is written, that Abraham had two sons, the one by a bondmaid, the other by a freewoman.*

But he who was of the bondwoman was born after the flesh; but he who was born of the freewoman was by promise. Now all these things are an allegory; these two women represent two covenants. One covenant's origin is Mount Sinai where Moses received the law (Moses is dead), and this covenant only bears children whose destiny is slavery: this is the woman Hagar. Now this Hagar stands for Mount Sinai in Arabia and she belongs in the same category with the present physical Jerusalem, for she is in bondage together with her children. But the Jerusalem above is free: this is the woman Sarah. Now this Sarah bears children that are not by physical descent, as was Ishmael, but like Isaac born in virtue of promise. But as then, he that was born after the flesh persecuted him that was born after the Spirit, even so it is now. Nevertheless what does the scripture say? Get rid of the women of slavery and her son; for the son of the bondwoman will not be heir with the son of Sarah, for she represents that Jerusalem that is not natural, but supernatural.

Amplified! 1st Corinthians 3:16 *Know ye not that*

your bodies are the temple of the Holy Spirit?

Hebrews 10:19-22 *Therefore, brothers, since we have confidence to enter the Most Holy Place by the blood of Jesus, by a new and living way open for us through the curtain, that is, his body ...let us draw near to God with a sincere heart in full assurance of faith.*

So, the answer to our 2nd question. Where is the temple and the altar?

Today, believers represent that city, their bodies are the temple thereof and their heart is the altar which is God's dwelling place; this is the city not made with hands that Abraham was looking for.

Questions 3 & 4: Who were the healers in the Bible and what did they use for medicine?

As believers, we have been quite ignorant of something that the priests were well aware of when people came to them for help. They understood the connection between the soul and the body's reaction to it. I am happy, however, to say that we are beginning to be awakened to this connection. The priests understood this basic principle: "There is most assuredly, a connection between the soul and body that affects our health". Priests dealt, not only with the healing of the body, but the soul of man as well.

Understanding that during Jesus's life He was under the Old Covenant, He confirms the priest's role when He healed ten lepers. They were healed as they went and Jesus sent them to the priests because under the Levitical priesthood the law allowed only the priests to say a person was healed.

Luke 17:12-14 *And as he was going into one village, He was met by ten lepers, who stood at a distance. And they raised up their voices and called, "Jesus, Master, take pity and have mercy on us"! And when He saw them He said to them;*

Go (at once) and show yourselves to the priests. And as they went they were cured and made clean.

Leviticus 14:1-3: *And the Lord spoke to Moses, This shall be the law of the leper on the day he is to be pronounced clean: he shall be brought to the priest to examine him and behold if the plague of leprosy be healed in the leper, etc.*

A great deal of Matthew, Mark, Luke and John were written about people who were still living under the Old Covenant, as it wasn't until the resurrection that the New Covenant was made known. It was not until 70 AD that the sacrifices stopped completely at the destruction of the temple.

So how did the priests minister healing? They used the same principle throughout the Bible that we see in the New Covenant. They used oil with prayer. Only we lost the significance of the oil! We lost the significance of therapy! We have a vision for Divine Health, not just the need for healing, and the reality of it is that God, in His Infinite Grace, has provided more than His miracles for healing. He provided medicine; His medicine. We love it when God heals instantly. We desire it, but what about those who are not healed in this manner. Mostly, we have counseled them into condemnation, sorry to say. It has been out of our ignorance that we have done this. Let us change this. Let us encourage one another into health and wholeness. Let us teach "All" that God has given us, not just a portion: Miracles and Therapy! Again, Ezekiel 47:12 – *"Along the bank of the river, on this side and that, will grow all kinds of trees used for food. Their leaves will not wither, and their fruit will be for food, and their leaves shall be for medicine".* Trees and leaves did not change when the law changed!

A priest's ministry then, is not only to the soul of man, but also to the body. This is why John stated in 3rd John 2: Beloved, I wish above ALL things that you may prosper and be in health, even as your <u>soul</u> prospers. We understand now why ministering to the soul and healing the body is the calling of a priest? Today, you are that priest; today, you are that healer, today you care for your temple as well as helping another. Today you can use Bible oils and prayer from "God's Medicine Cabinet"! It is a privilege and a responsibility to be a part of this priesthood as we come to Him. Together, we can "Seize the Kingdom on Healing".

CHAPTER 5 – The Best of the Best

There can be no doubt! If you have read this book with understanding, you now comprehend the best natural thing God gave us for healing and the health of our bodies, is Bible oils.

The world would like to divert our attention from Bible oils and focus on a worldly aspect of oils giving them the recognition that only God deserves. We want to honor God by recommending the oils that are giving God the glory.

No one has any right to decisions about your health but YOU! Let no one ever tell you differently. This entire effort to get this information to you is not about business. It is about YOU!... We offer the following for your consideration as you make life choices concerning your own needs. Synergistic blends of Bible oils have proven to be of tremendous benefit as the effect of the blends are greater than the total effect of an individual oil.

So, now we have available to us some blended oils mentioned in the Bible. Acknowledging God as the One who created them for our benefit, they are the best of the best. To see the body of Christ walk in divine healing and health is within our reach. Glory to God!

You can use the following format to profile yourself and what you may choose to use for your own health regime. Following this list, we offer some testimonies from those who have used these Bible oils.

****

12 BASIC – FOUNDATIONAL BIBLE OILS

****

FRANKINCENSE: Anti-septic, disinfectant, digestive, diuretic, and is used as a sedative as well as so many other medical benefits. It was included in this oil combination especially for supporting the nervous system. Supports the nervous system, and relaxes the body when eating.

MYRRH: Myrrh is especially used here for its powerful antioxidant effect. Topically, myrrh has been used to treat muscular pain. Myrrh can help decrease swelling (inflammation) and kill bacteria. Documented uses and benefits of myrrh are many...to name a few; bronchitis, diabetes, cancer, viral hepatitis, fungal infections (Candida, eczema, ringworm, athletes foot, vaginal thrush), tooth and gum conditions, skin conditions (wrinkles, stretch marks, chapped, cracked skin), diarrhea, dysentery, hyperthyroidism, and ulcers. Works on our thyroid and endocrine, immune and nervous systems. Regulates moods, growth and development, tissue function, metabolism, sexual function and reproductive processes. Balances out hormonal levels.

SANDALWOOD: Calms the mind, soothes stress, nervous tension, and uplifts the mood. It is used for skin conditions, cold sores, viral infections, such as herpes, wrinkles AND scars...also an excellent anti-septic and anti-inflammatory.

CINNAMON BARK: Balances blood sugars, minimizes inflammation that combats infections. Removes blood impurities, a natural immune system booster, a natural anti-viral, anti-fungal remedy that combats bacterial infections; Protects the stomach from ulcers, protects the heart and blood vessels. Kills warts, worms and eases digestive complaints.

SPIKENARD: Sedates inflammation in the digestive and nervous system, sedates irritations, nervous afflictions, convulsions, depression, stress and feelings of anxiety, anger, and panic.

HELICHRYSUM OIL: A nervine. Strengthens and protects the nervous system; as such it is anti-spasmodic giving quick relief from spasms. Reduces anxiety, lowers stress levels.

CASSIA: Alleviates mental fatigue, sexual disorders, and depression.

CYPRESS: Used for urinary, liver, cardiovascular, muscular and joint health.

LEMON: Invigorating, promoting a deep sense of well-being. Adjusts our pH levels, and lowers blood pressure. Cleaner for the lymphatic system. Gives energy and vivacity to the body and the mind. Improves mental accuracy and concentration. Diminishes mental exhaustion and lethargy.

PEPPERMINT: Ability to treat indigestion, respiratory problems, headache, nausea, fever, stomach and bowel spasms, and urinary tract infections. Fights fatigue, very stimulating, enhances the capability to concentrate, and brings clarity of thoughts and decisions, helps with insomnia, distress, tension, anxiousness, lethargy and / or vertigo (light-headedness). In addition: Helps with weight loss.

CLOVE: Indigestion, cough, asthma, headache, stress and blood impurities. Has antiseptic properties useful for wounds, cuts, scabies, athlete's foot, fungal infections, bruises, and prickly heat.

CEDARWOOD: Alleviates stress, calms and purifies, reduces stress and tension. Calming, purifying properties. Good for hair loss, acne and eczema. Has anti-fungicidal properties!

Application of oils: Apply a few drops of oil unto the right thumb and index finger and put to your nose and breathe in and out deeply 8-9 times, 3-4 times a day. It is hoped the aroma will be pleasing as the benefits of oils as they mix with your blood and very rapidly reach every cell in your body. As the blood brain barrier is penetrated, the oxygen you breathe in, along with the oils reach deeply into your very being. Look for a change in your outlook on life and a sense of well-being.

ANOTHER BIBLE OIL

HYSSOP: Purifies from addictions and destructive habits; It metabolizes fat, increases perspiration for detoxification, and helps with emotional balance.

TESTIMONIES

I have been mostly bed ridden. I have only been able to make quick trips to the store to get a few items (just in and out) when absolutely necessary. I have been in so much pain in my back, legs, feet, and toes. I would get up from bed and get a drink of water and then get right back into bed to prop my feet up. I have not slept all through the night in more than 7 years. I have tried everything to try to help myself. I have gone to Specialists and went through all the needles and electric tests. The pain of the needles should have been excruciating. The Dr. even made me bleed and still I felt no additional pain. The problem with my situation is that I am in so much pain all the time, but can't tell if I step on anything and will trip if anything like a vacuum cord is in my path....it's been terrible. A constant numbness, tingling, burning, red feet, hurting like someone is hitting my legs and feet with a hammer. It's like my legs below my knees feel like they have been dipped in cement and the cement has hardened. The Specialist diagnosed me with having Neuropathy and as being permanently disabled and issued me a State Disability Pass for parking and going to parks. I a combination of oils on my feet and noticed a real difference in 15 minutes. I finally felt relief. I sleep all through the night using these oils. I put them on my feet and lower back and there has been a definite improvement. I studied these oil's and the Frankincense and Myrrh Oil's represent Christ. The way it is harvested is like Jesus Christ death, burial, and resurrection. I went to the Ocean yesterday, but would not have been able to do that without using some combination of oil's that were given to me as a gift from my Mother-in-law, for prayers, forgiveness, and Jesus Christ Love and Compassion to me. It's been so nice to have something to help soothe the tightness and burning sensations. It has helped relieve the pain so I can walk a little longer. It's an AMAZING gift God has given us and I THANK Him for them. I hope the oils get known because people need them. Now that I have tried them and felt relief, I don't want to be without them.....THEY REALLY ARE THAT GOOD. I truly have tried all the Dr's medicines, all the over-the-counter remedies, and all the friends and relatives suggestions and NOW have finally been truly blessed by using the bible oils. THANKS A MILLION. Robert/ USA.

■■■

I have been using the oils and I am the author of this book. I wanted to share my personal testimony because of the many trials I faced with insomnia. I hope no one ever has to go through 30 years of the accuser yelling in their ear that God doesn't love them. Because He gives His beloved sleep and I could not sleep, I faced that accusation nightly. Of course I tried everything from pharmaceuticals to everything natural I could find. Pharmaceuticals were a waste of time and taxing to my body, and although I believed in the natural things I used, they did not help me. I have finally found a place of rest at night and the knot that has been in my chest from all the anxiety it created, is gone. Bonnie / USA

****

My name is John. I use some blended oils. I have been using them for 2 months for weight loss and it is not so much that I have lost a LOT of weight, but I have lost one belt size. I had a piece of lemon pie the other night, which has always been my favorite, and I didn't really like it. I do not have the cravings for the sweets anymore. Phooey! HA, HA, HA! John / from Arizona.

****

I use the oils for pain. I work for "Dress Barn", a ladies fashion store in Phoenix, AZ. I am 78 so my arms get to hurting from lifting the clothes, especially around the rotary cuffs in my shoulders. My sciatic nerves that run along my legs also give me a real challenge. But, the bible oils get me through the day. They really do alleviate the pain, plus I like the restorative qualities of the bible oils. I rub it all over my upper arms and find that it takes the pain out from between my shoulders and upper arms. It works anywhere on my body that I have used it. Marilyn / from AZ

****

Being of true sound mind and body, truthfully testify that a combination of bible oils definitely relieve the tingling and pain in my feet. I officiate baseball and fast pitch games every year. The ointment provides the comfort I need to be able to rest and sleep after each ballgame. I understand that it is not only restorative, but also prevents the nerves from dying in my feet. I am very thankful to have been introduced to these oils. Dan/ from Arizona

****

I received a gift of a combination of oils from my mother and I am so thankful to God and to her for letting me have access to them. I have had a problem with anxiety and major panic attacks for quite some time that make me terribly sick, and at times wake me up at night, because I cannot breathe. The only way I could find some temporary relief, would be to open the outside door, and breathe in some fresh air. I sought my Doctor's help to no avail, searched the internet over, and tried everything I could to try to better myself. I steadily got worse and then began breathing heavily all day. Then the bible oils were introduced to me. I tried a mixture of oil's on my thumb and pointer finger, breathed it in my nose for a minute, and immediately the racing in my chest left. I breathed easier and lighter. The oils are amazing. I have been sleeping through the

Night with absolutely no problems with my breathing.

Now, whenever I feel anxious in the daytime, I will breath in the oil's and within minutes I start feeling much better. Some of the oils are a good remedy for relief when you are suffering with any kind of pain. Our pet dog has benefited from the oil's too. He has been to the vet multiple times for a cough he has suffered with since we got him 3 years ago. The veterinarian gives him an ear cream every time he goes in to get checked out. We decided to put oils on our dog's paws and in his ears and his coughing is almost cleared up. He coughed once last night and it was a quick short cough. It was not a long drawn out cough with a hack and a gag like it usually is. He is perked up like a puppy and seems so happy. I am really pleased with the way the Bible Oils help me to not feel anxious. God Bless You Abundantly. Renee / USA

■■

For oils email: abridgebuilder@gmail.com

Ph. 623-936-6204

LIST OF OILS OFFERED

CARRIER OILS

Carrier oils are also referred to as base oils. They are used to dilute single oils for application. Packaging in dark glass protects the integrity of each oil. This ensures that light does not disrupt each oils individual properties.

APRICOT – AVACADO – CAMELLIA – EVENING PRIMROSE – GRAPESEED – HAZELNUT – HEMP SEED – JOJOBA – MACAMIA – MEADOWFOAM – ROSEHIP – SESAME – SWEET ALMOND

Basic 12 SINGLE BIBLE OILS

Cassia – Cedarwood – Cinnamon Bark– Clove – Cypress– Frankincense– Helichyrsum – Lemon – Myrrh – Peppermint – Sandalwood – Spikenard

Others are available upon request at:

abridgebuilder@gmail.com

All Italics: BIBLE OILS

WORDS YOU MAY NOT BE FAMILIAR WITH:

LIMBIC: The center of emotions and memory in the brain.

MICROBES: Dangerous Fungus

ANTI-OXIDANT: A substance that inhibits oxidation

BALSAMS: An aromatic resinous substance, such as balm, exuded by various trees and shrubs and used as a base for certain fragrances and medical and cosmetic preparations.

NEURON: A specialized cell transmitting nerve impulses; a nerve cell.

NERVINE: Used to calm the nerves.

FREE RADICALS: An especially reactive atom or group of atoms that has one or more unpaired electrons; especially : one that is produced in the body by natural biological processes or introduced from an outside source – as tobacco smoke, toxins, or pollutants) and that can damage cells, proteins, and DNA by altering their chemical structure.